This Book Belongs To:

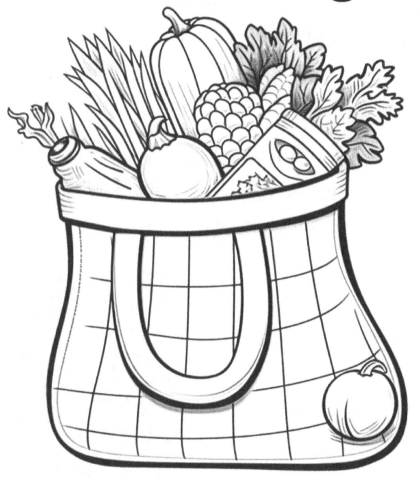

About Us

Brissa Ocean is an independent brand, that offers a world of creativity and artistic expression through a wide range of unique and captivating drawings.

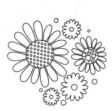

Our books are designed to provide you with an opportunity to disconnect, find tranquility, and rediscover the joy of creation.

Head on over to our Amazon Store for more:

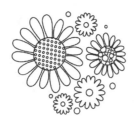

Thanks for adding a bit more color to the world!

 Brissa Ocean

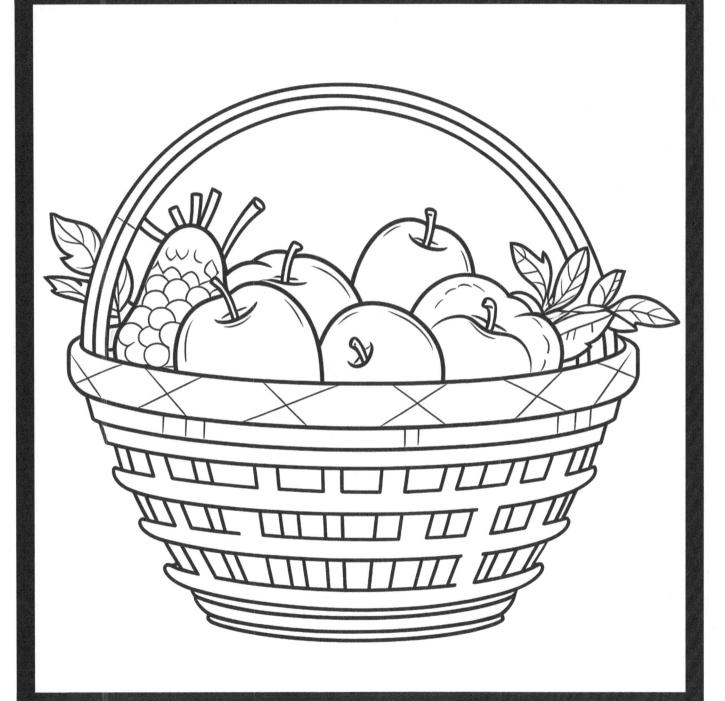

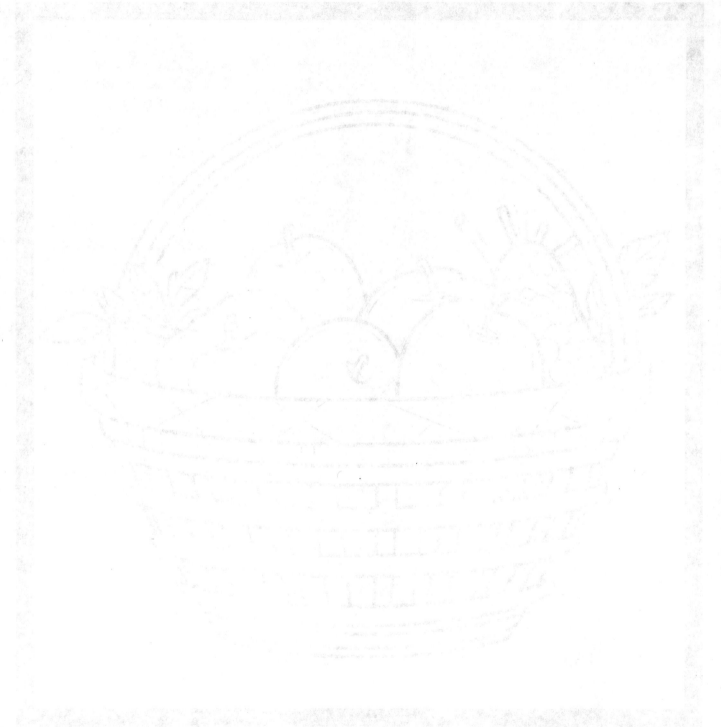

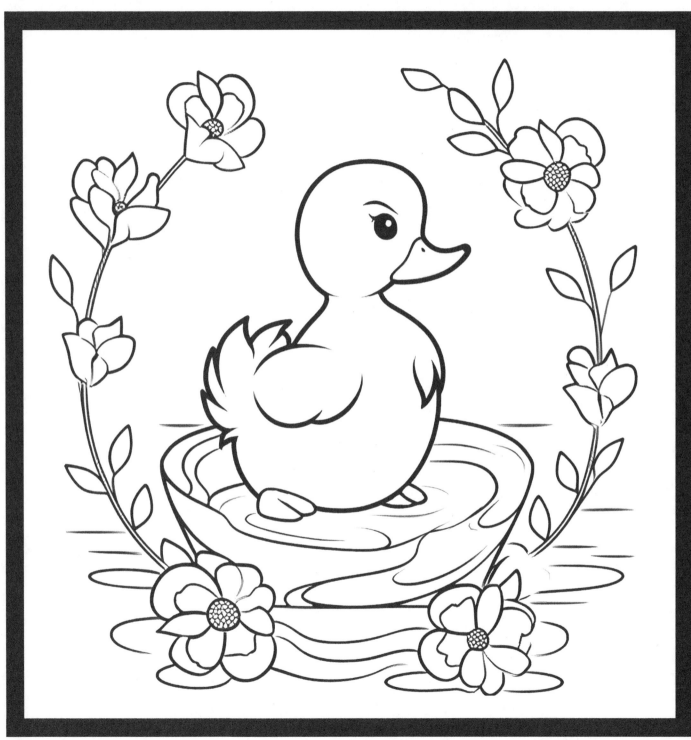

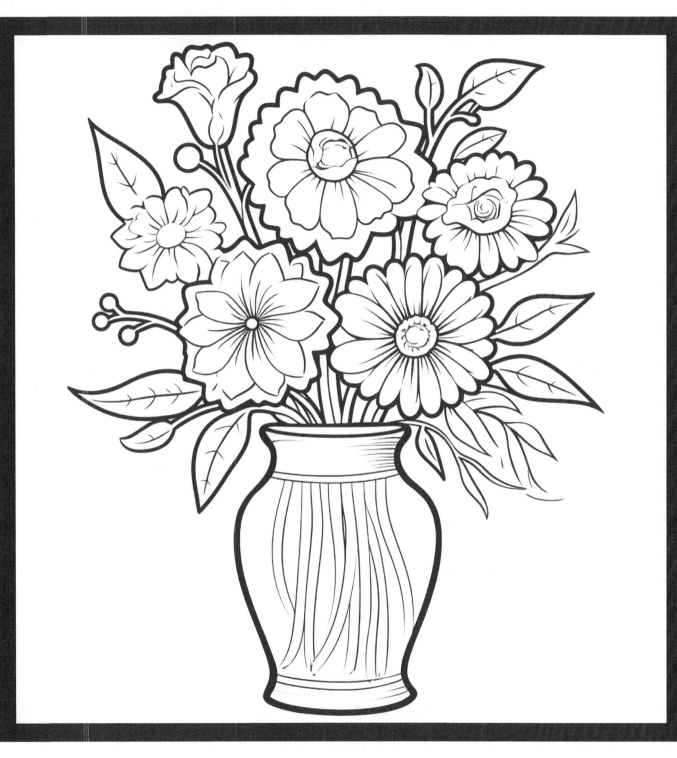

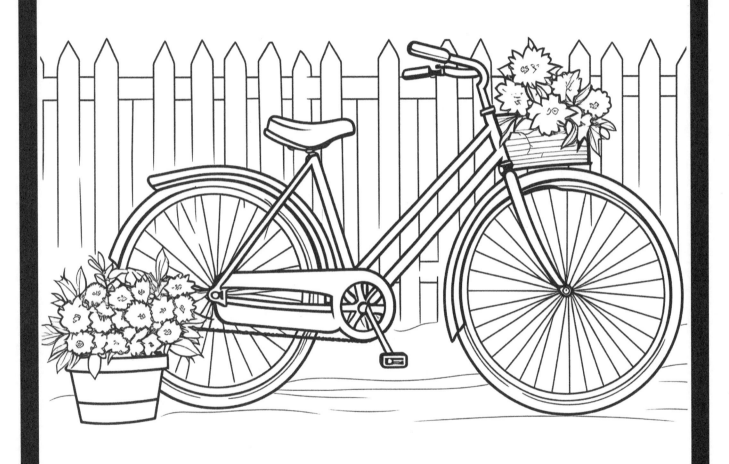

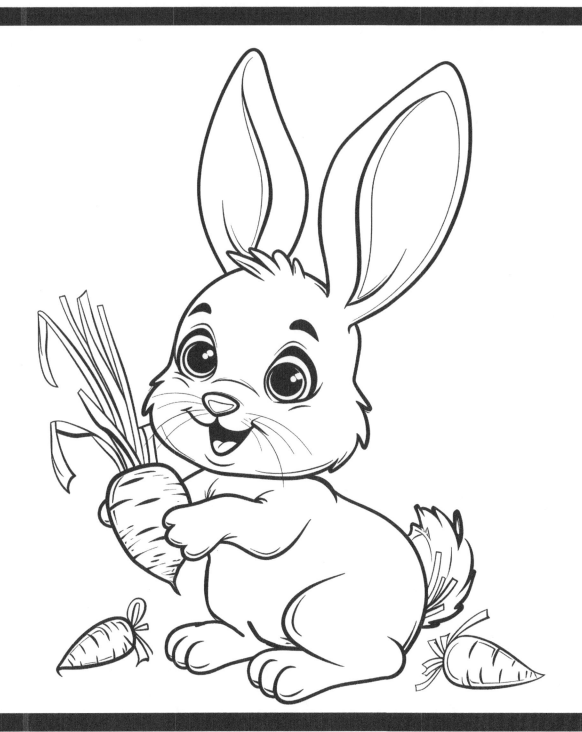

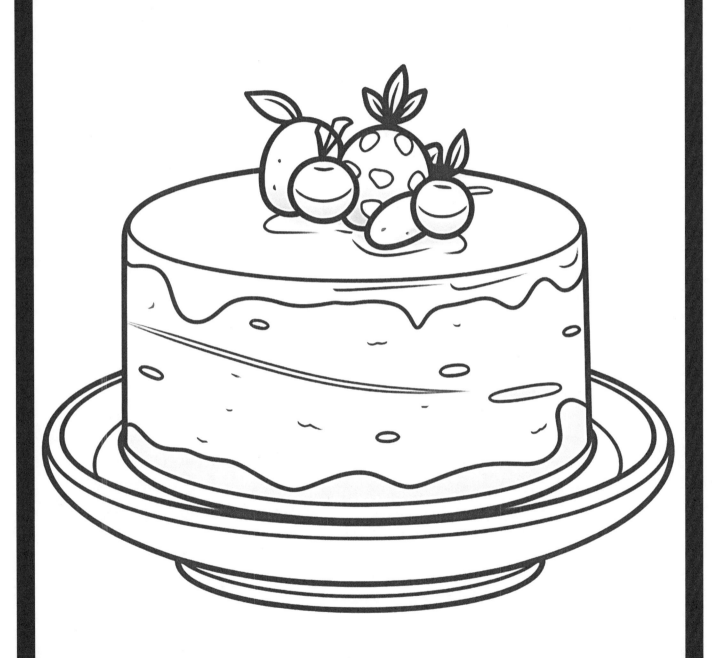

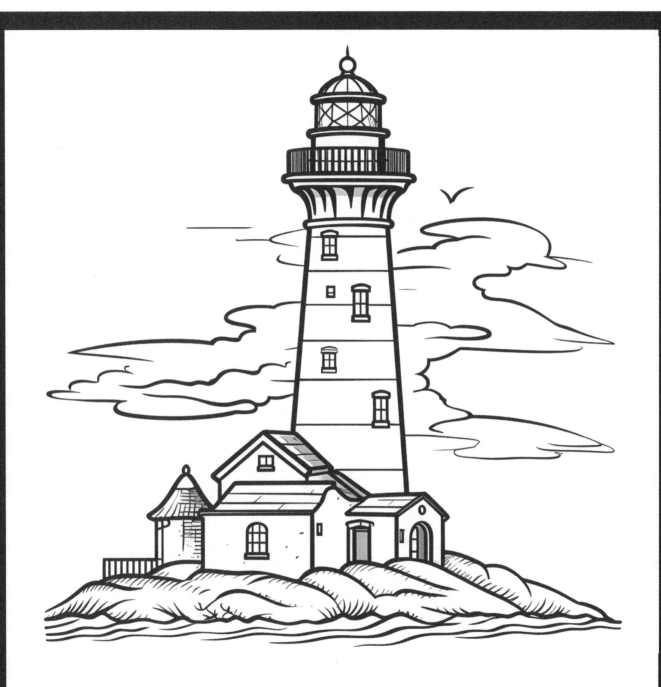

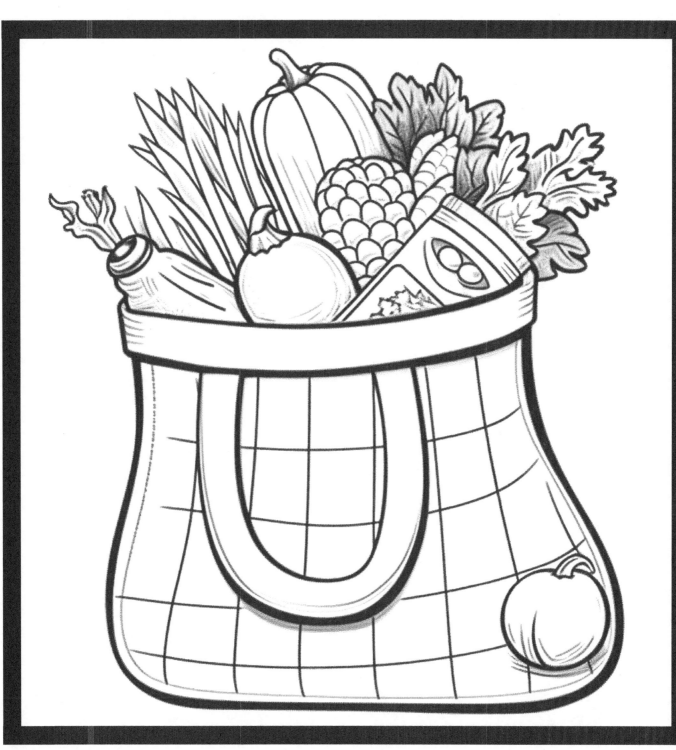

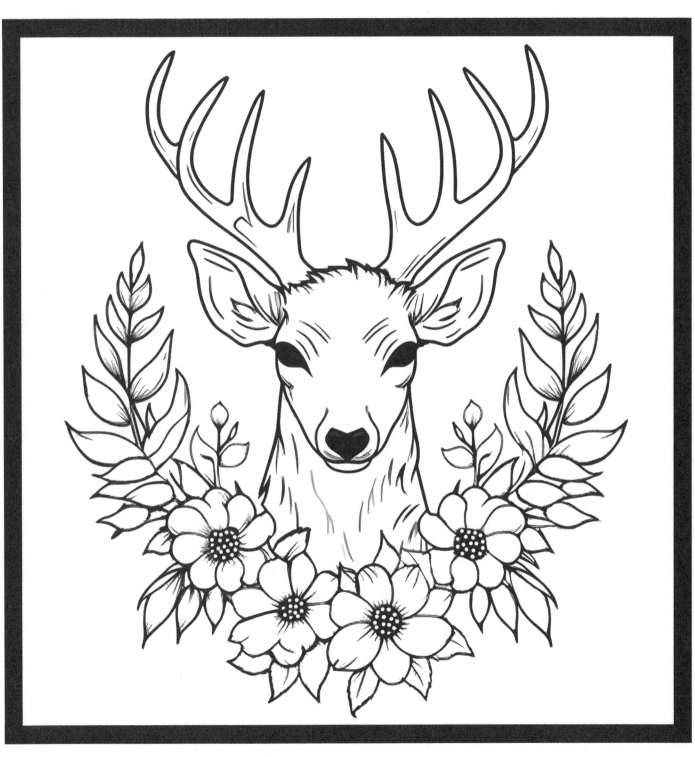

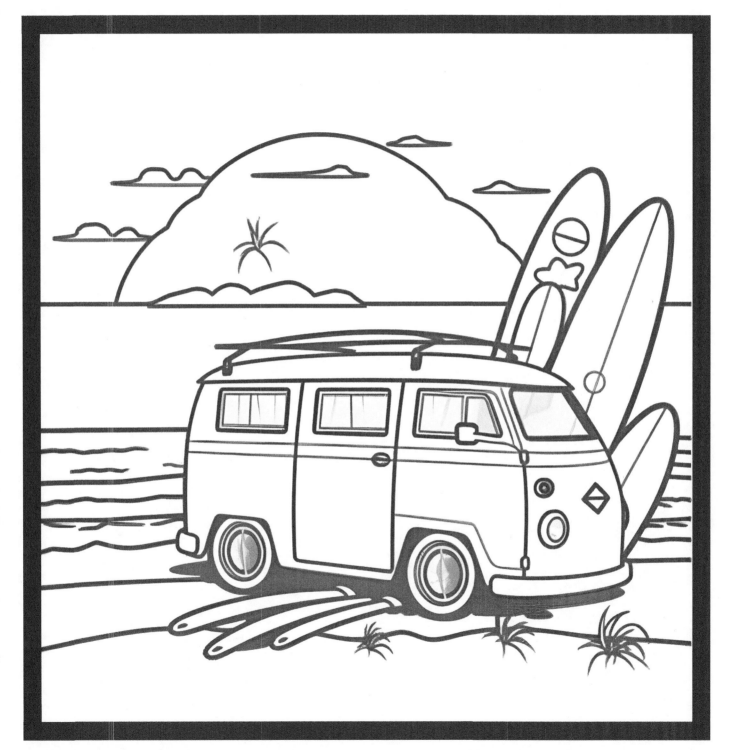

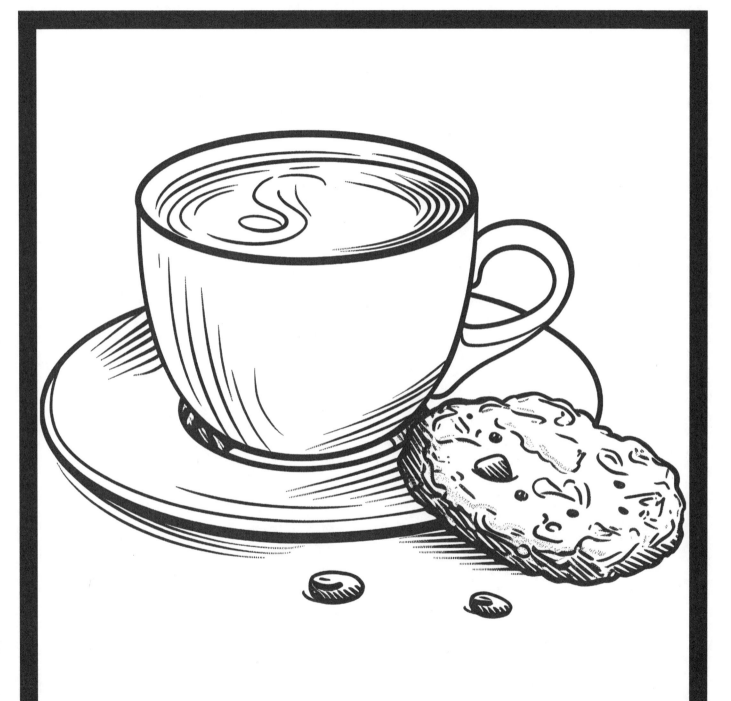

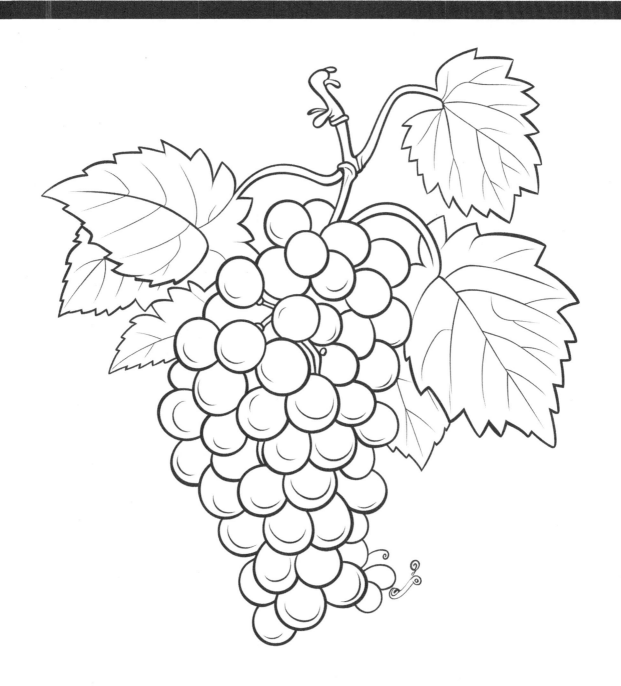

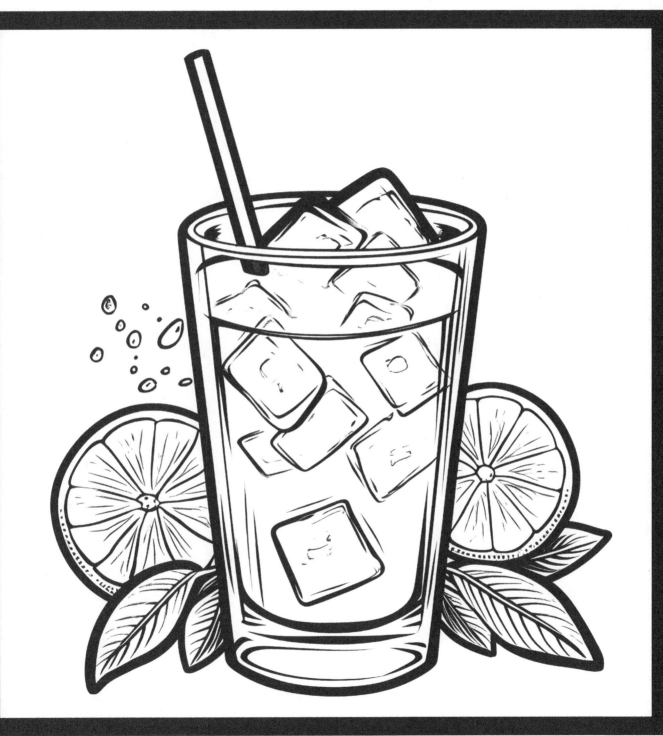

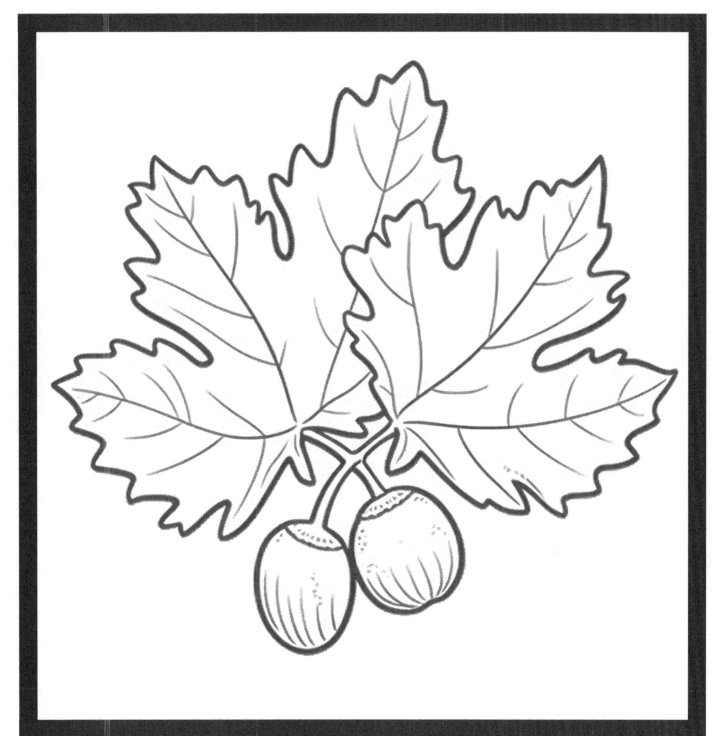

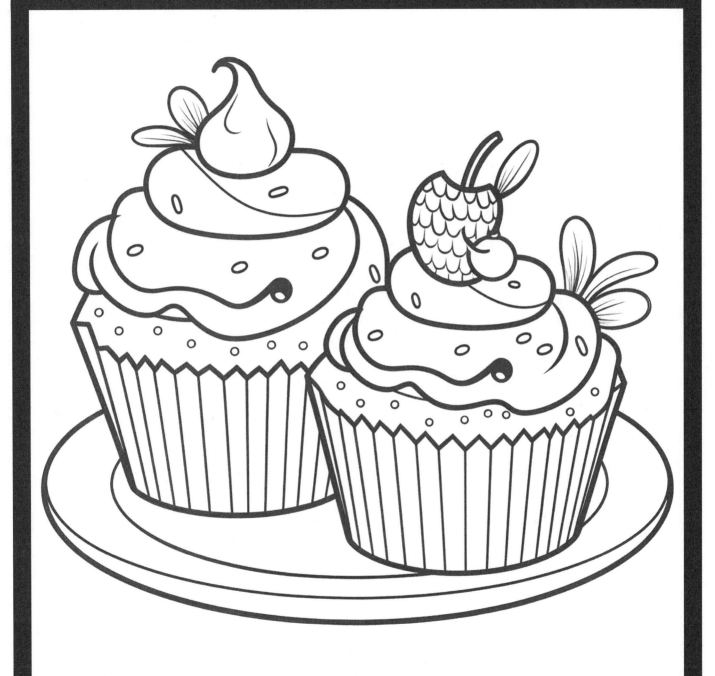

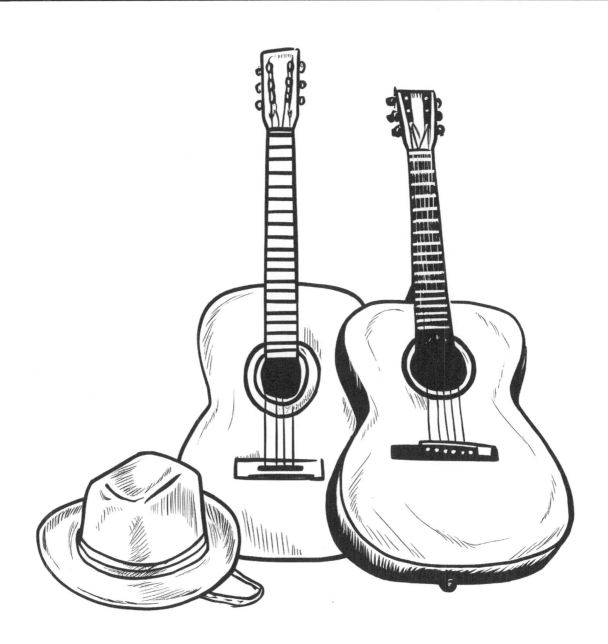

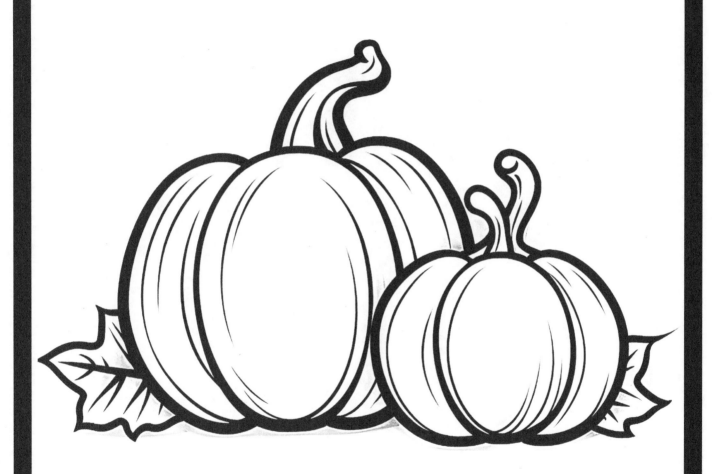

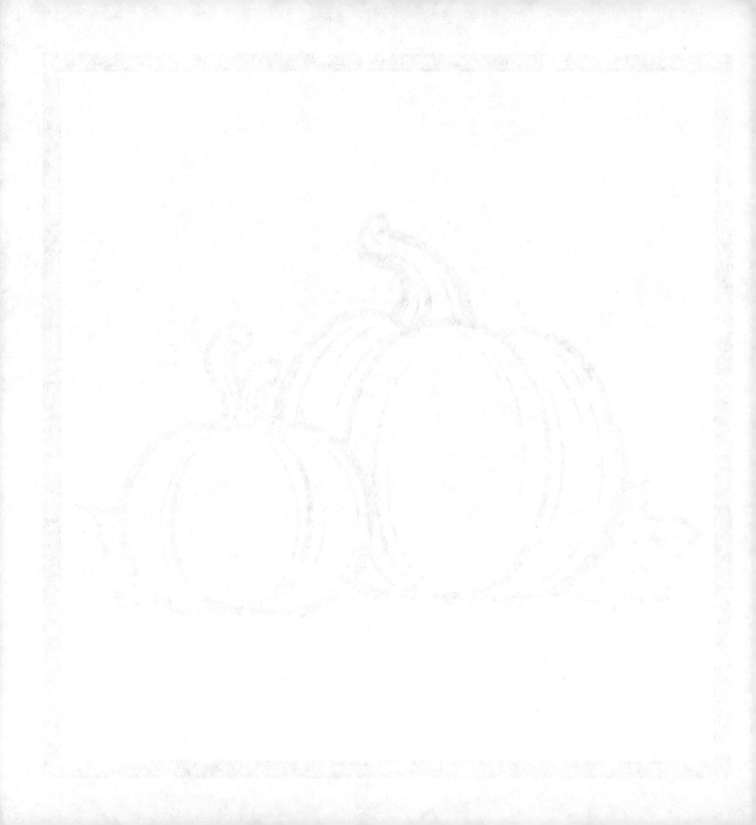

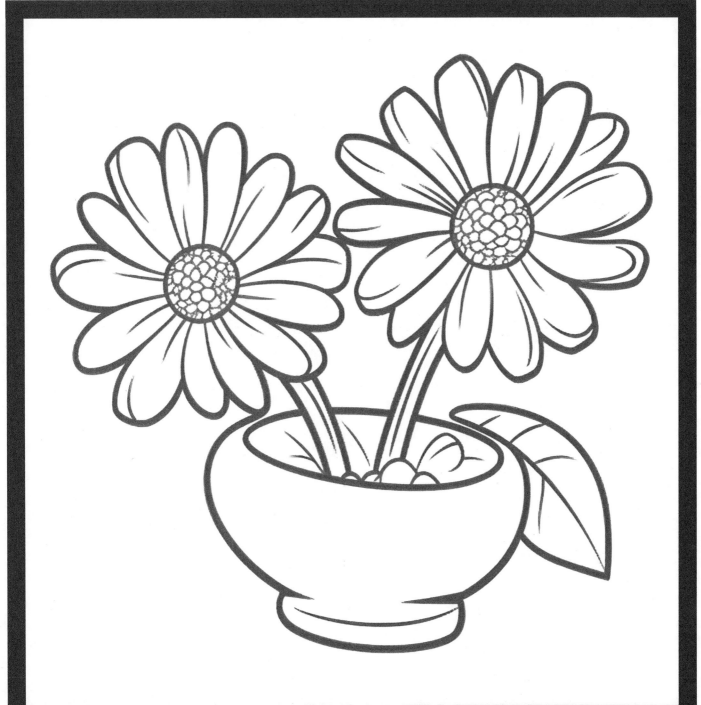

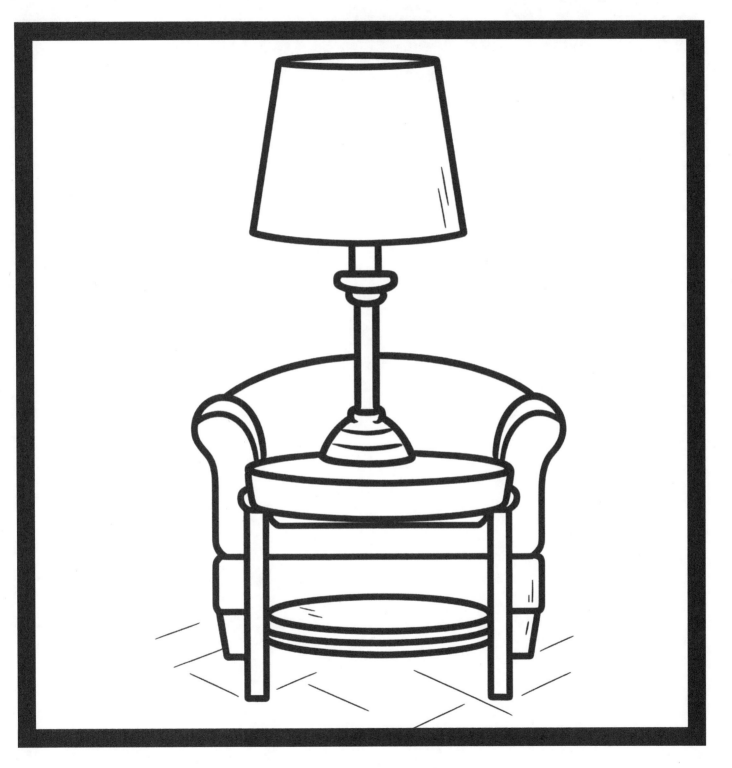

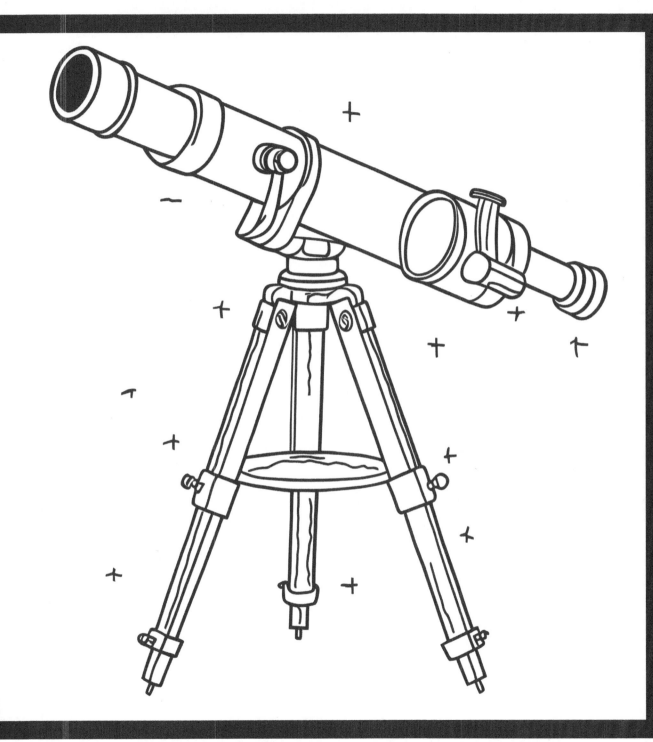

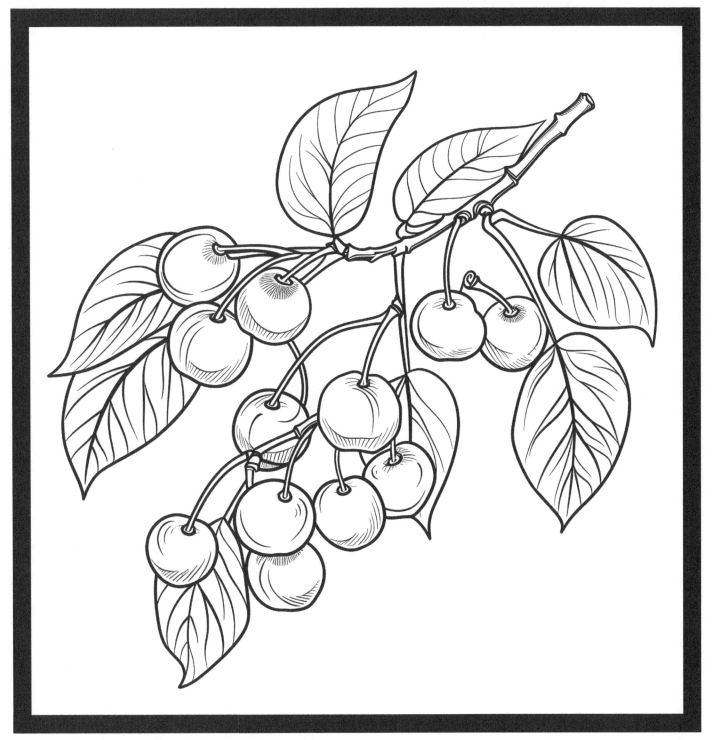

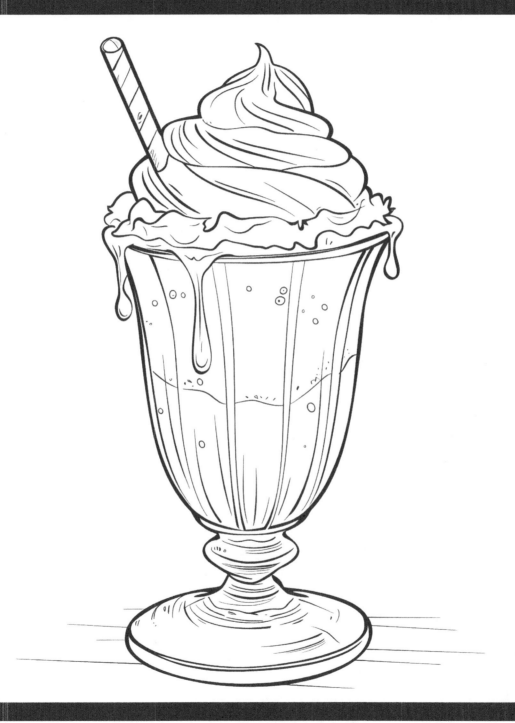

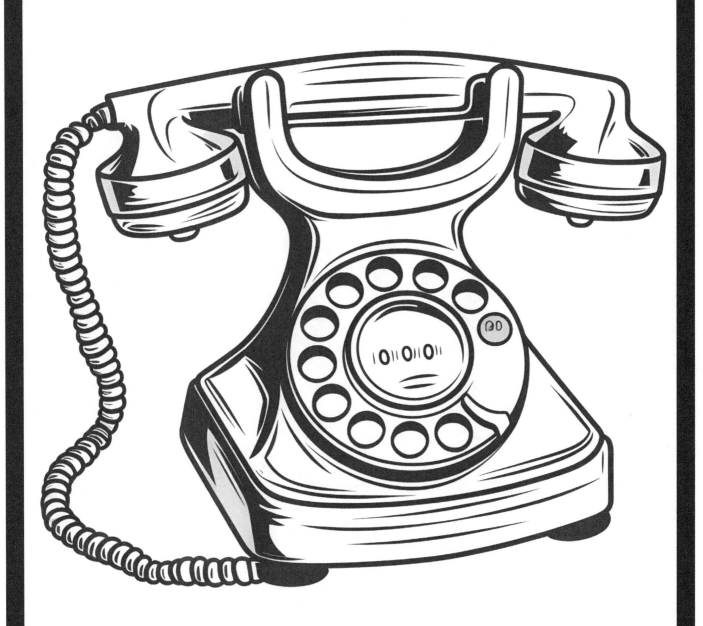

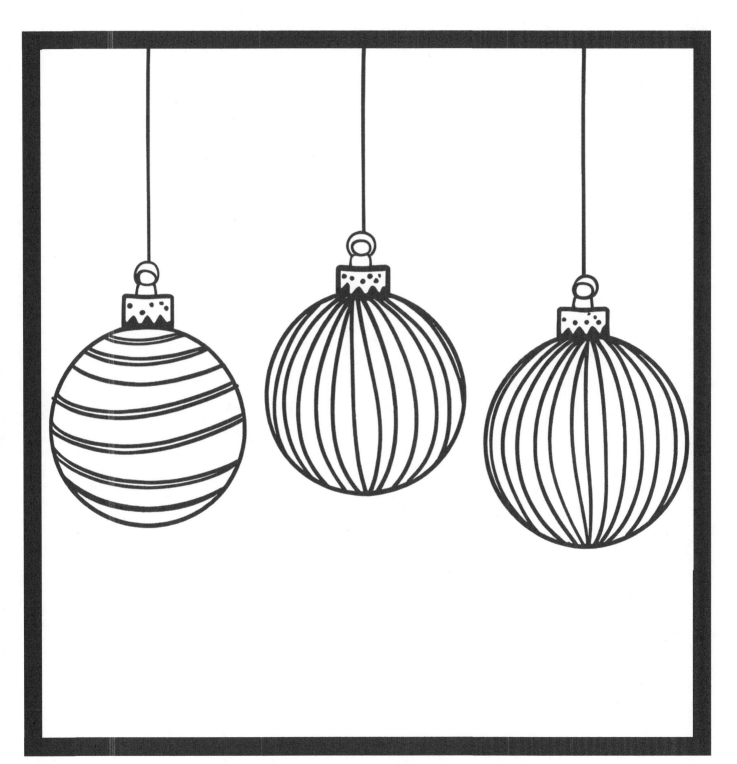

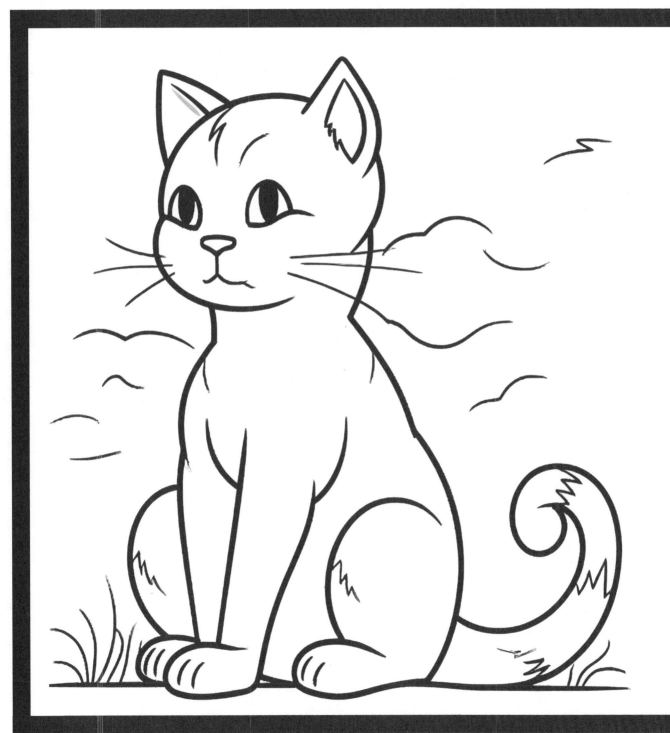

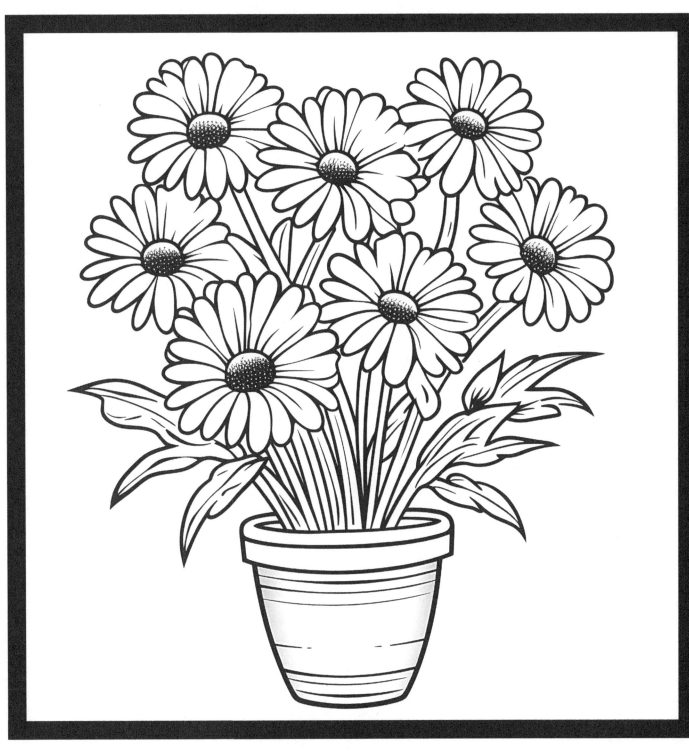

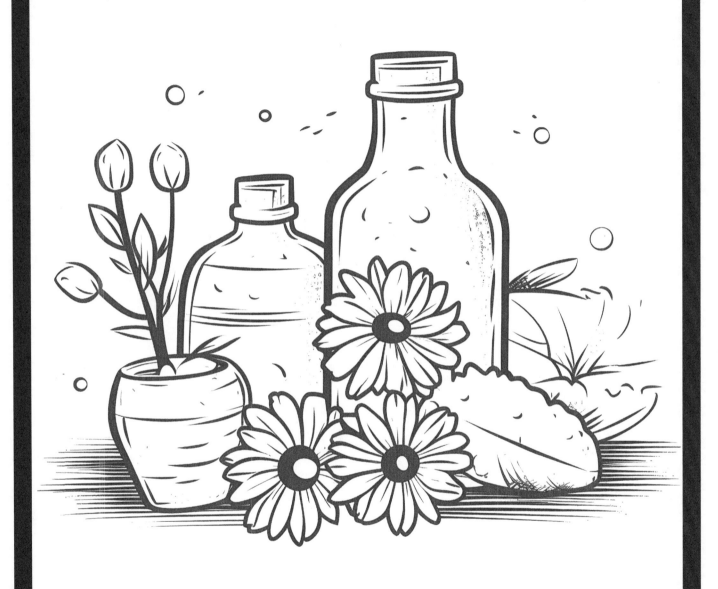

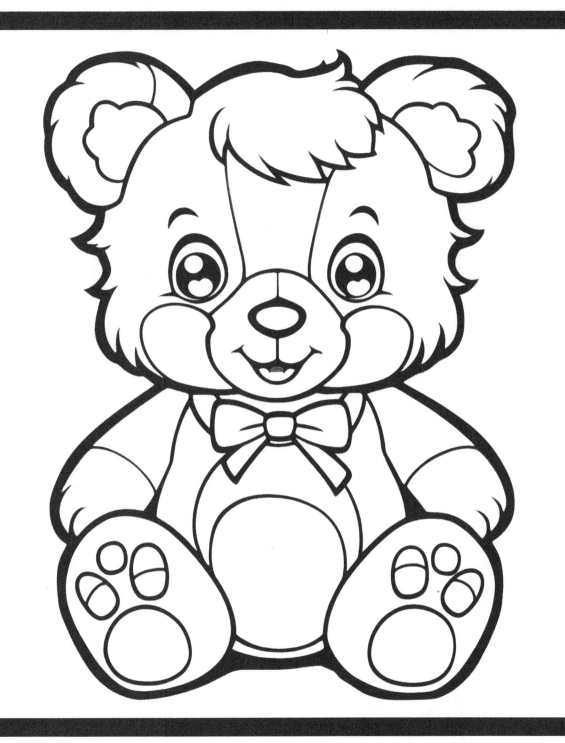

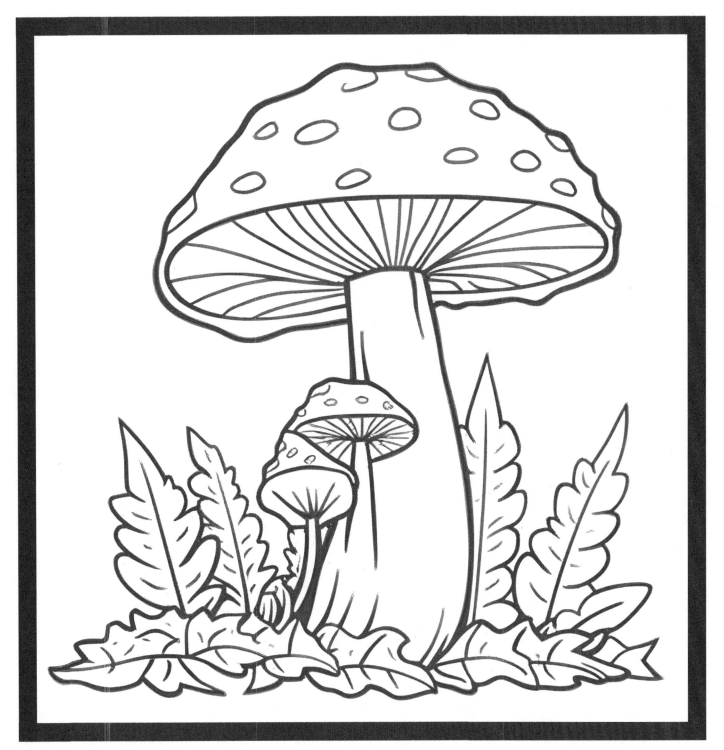

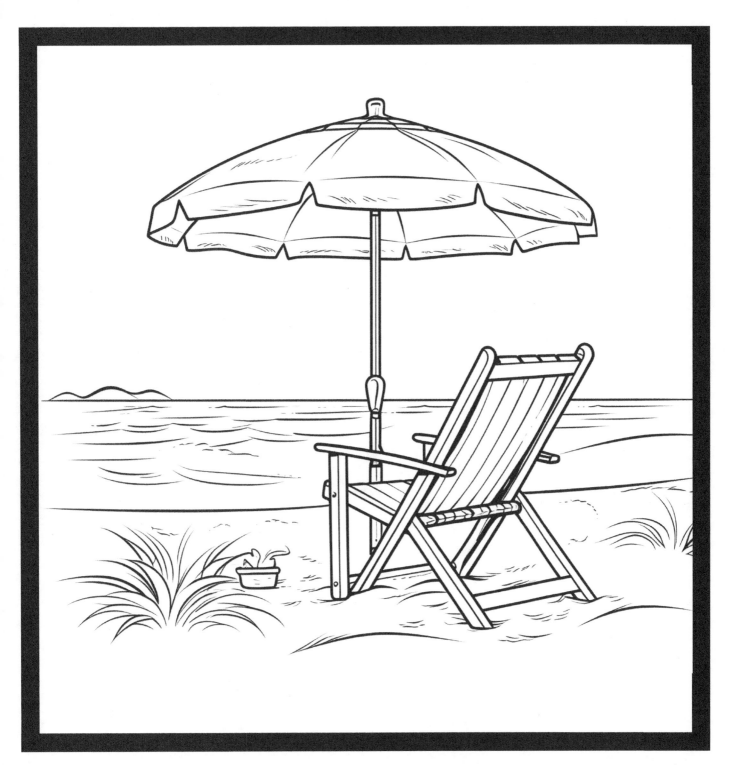

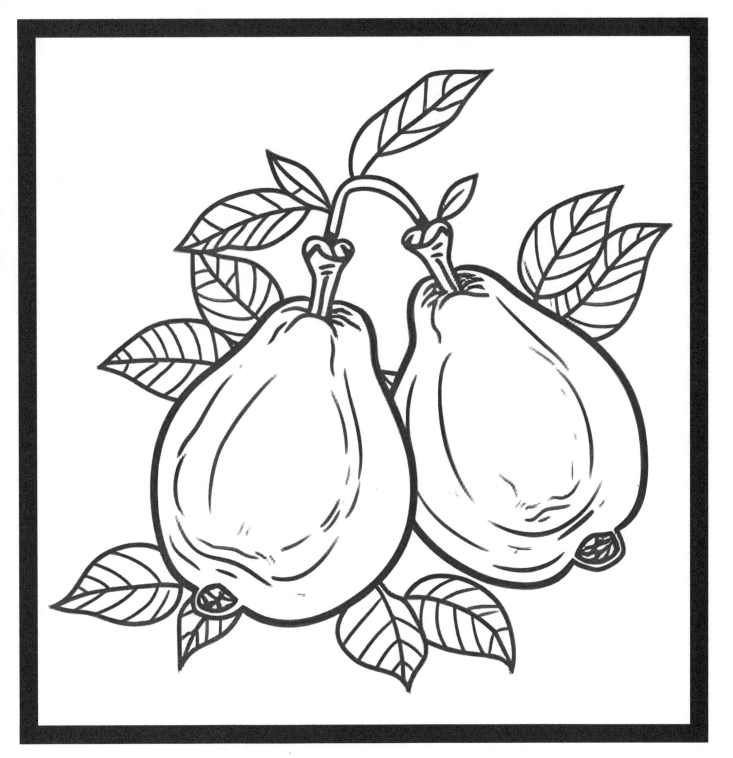

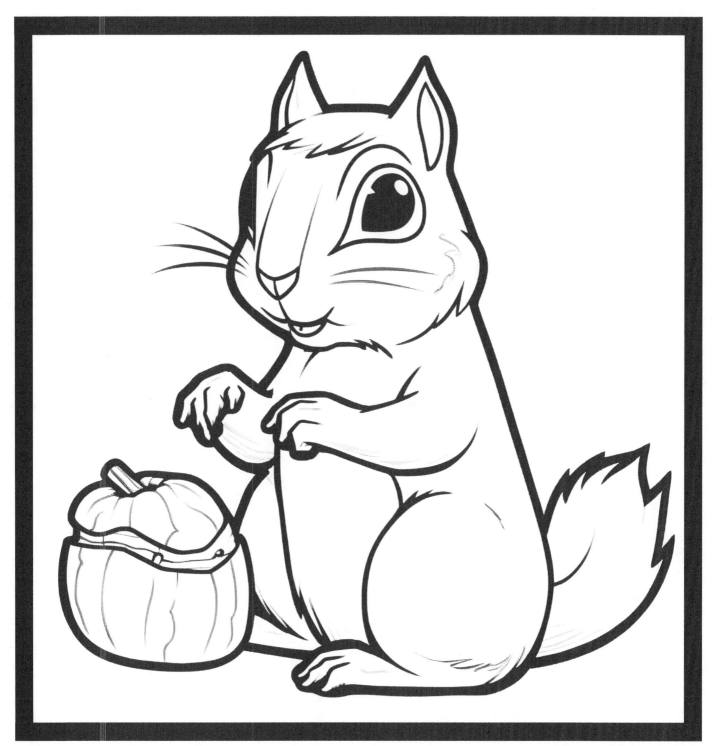

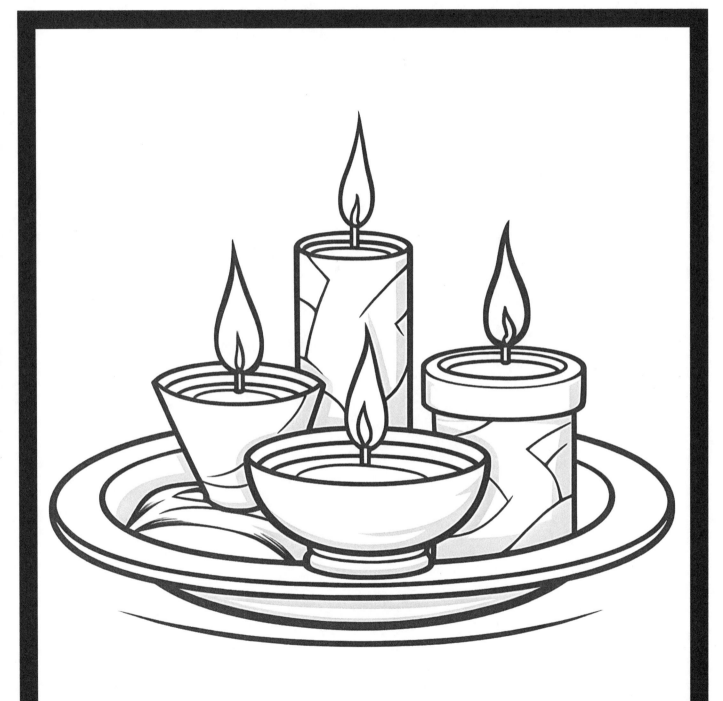

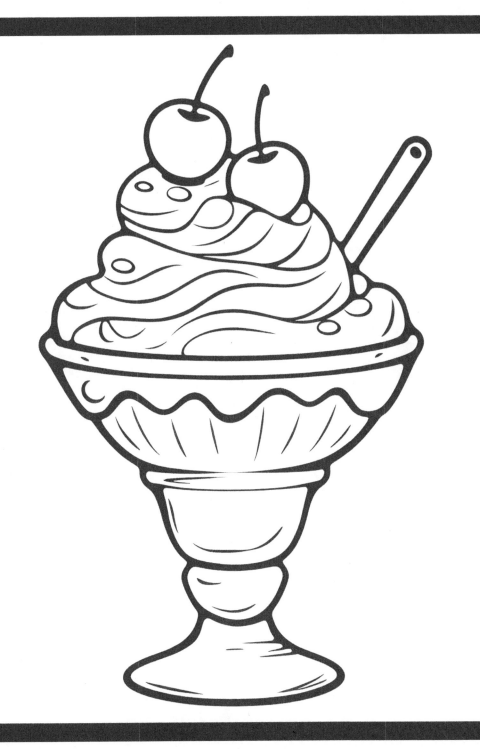

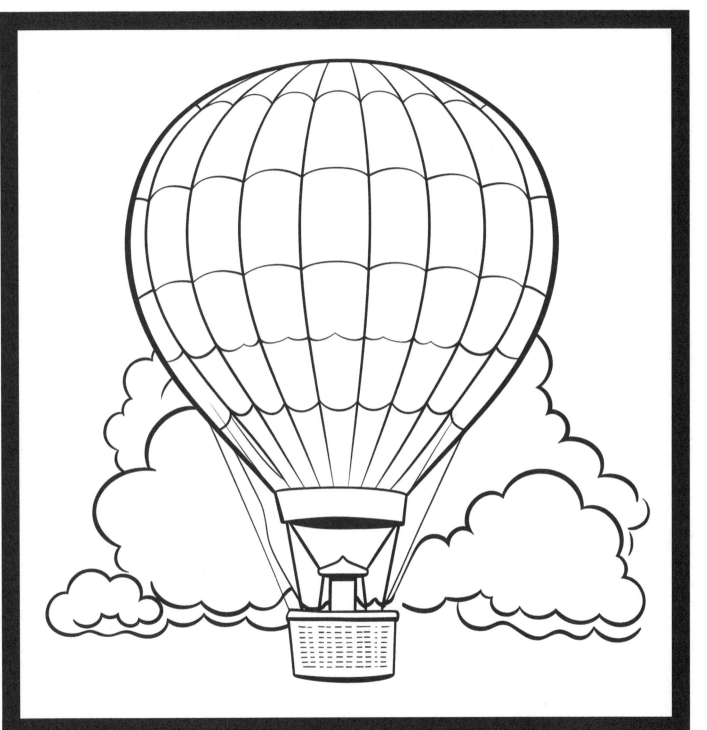

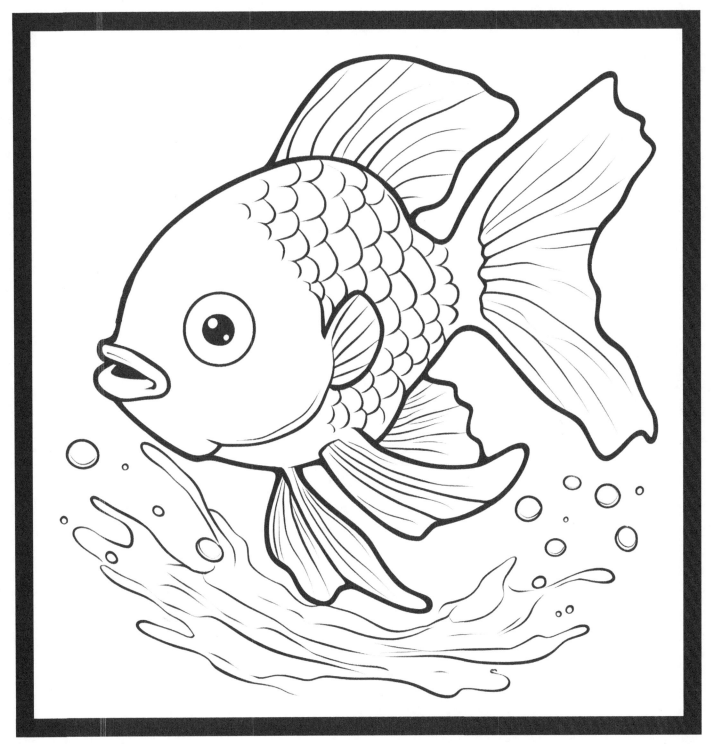

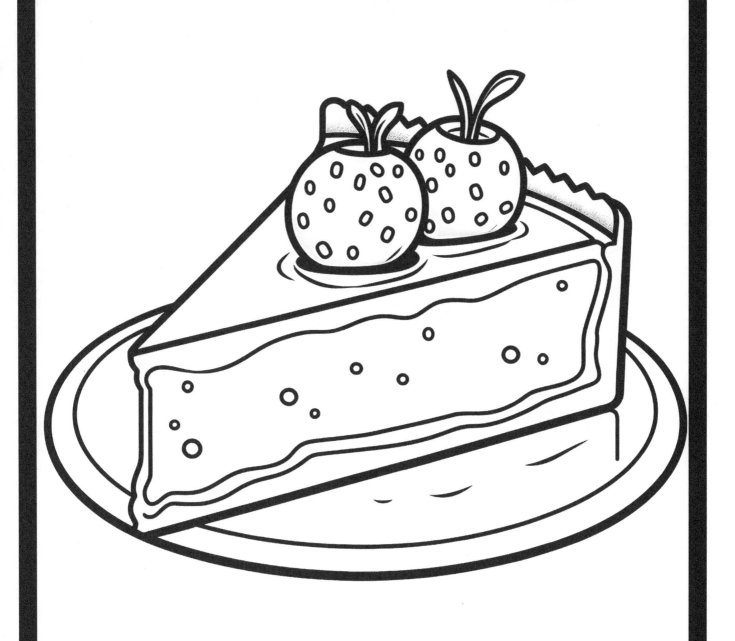

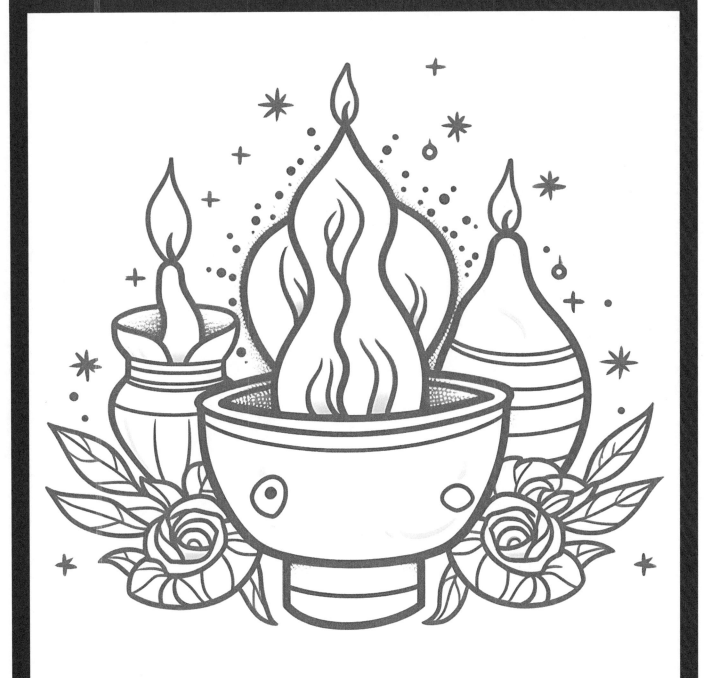

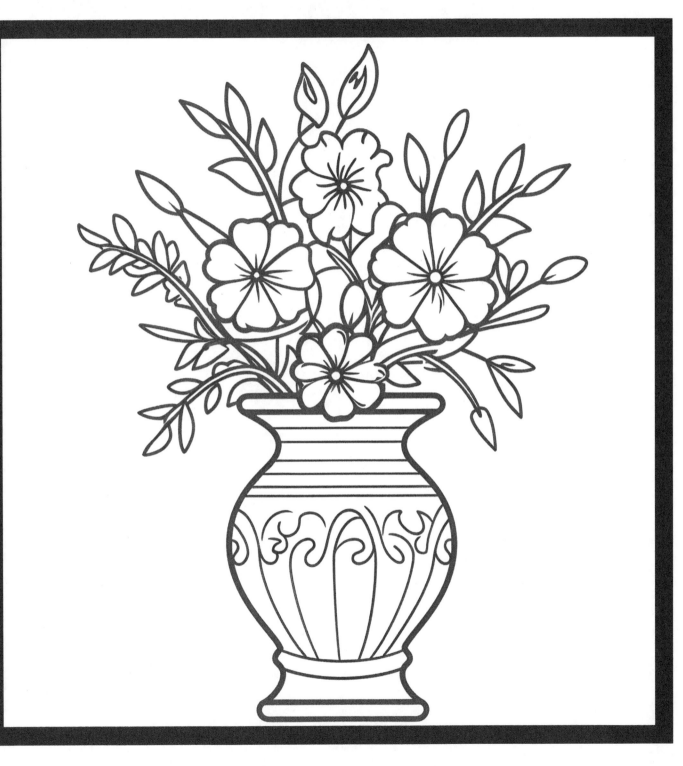

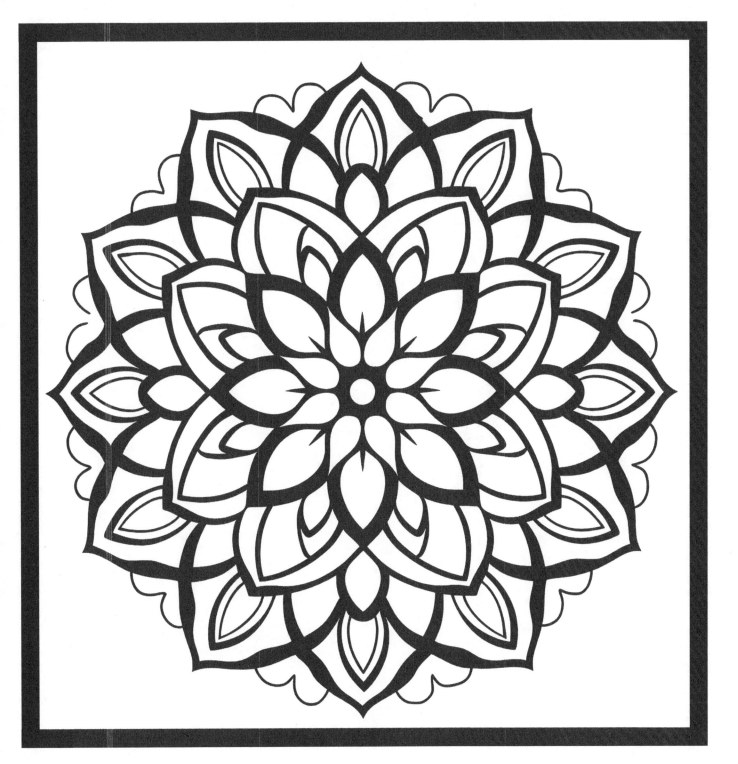

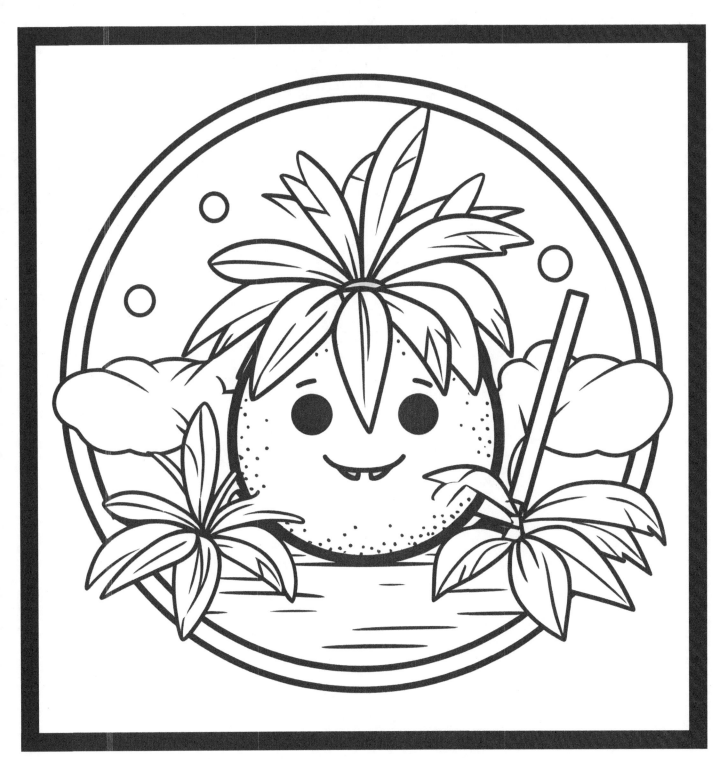

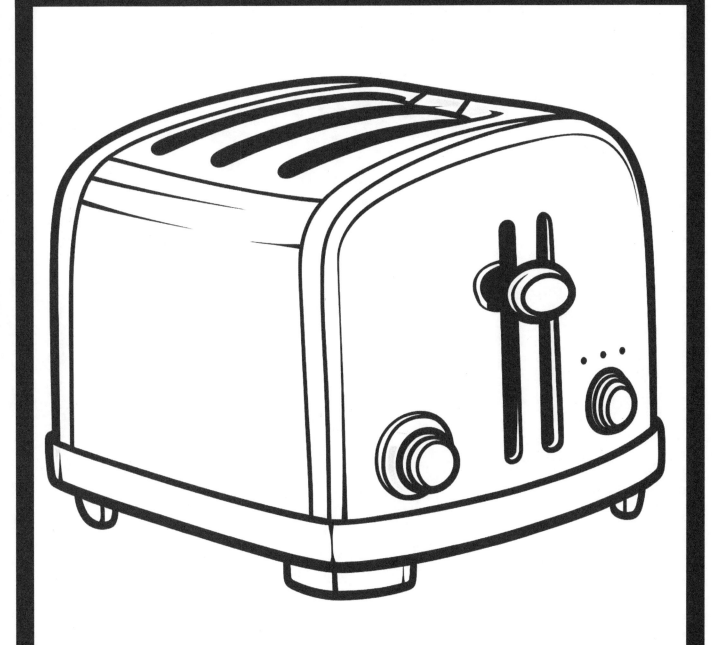

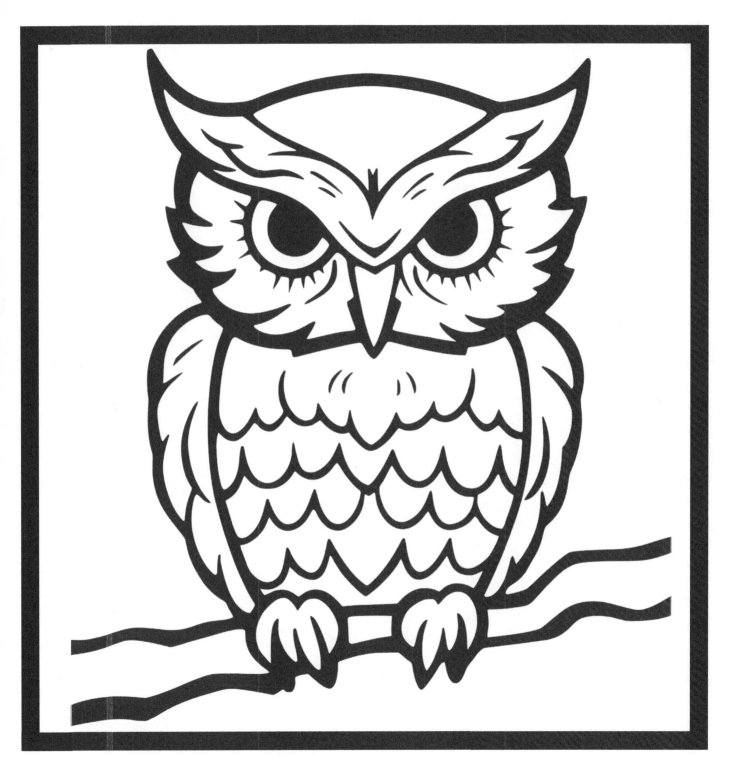

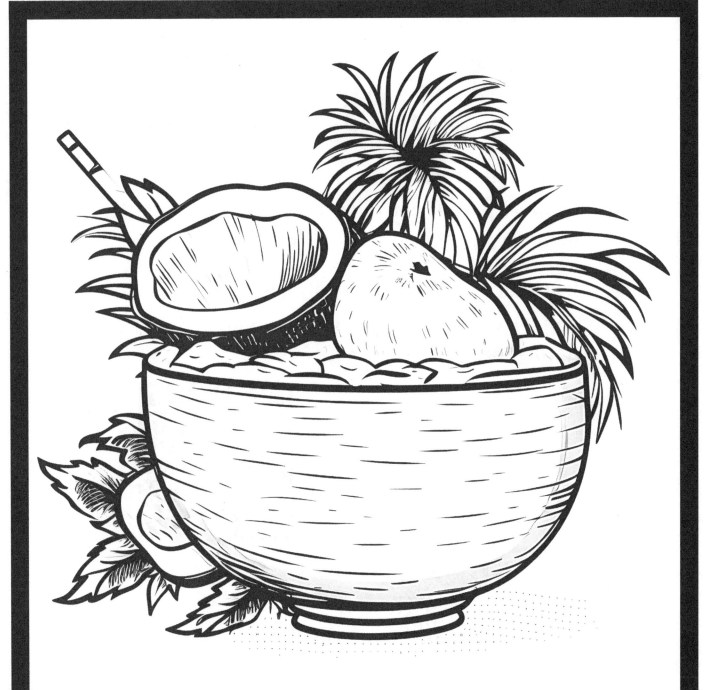

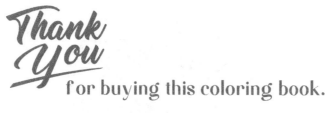 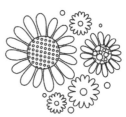

Thank You for buying this coloring book.

If you enjoyed your journey through these images, please consider taking a few minutes to leave a review.

It would mean the world to me, and I believe it can also help others find enjoyment in these pages.

This QR code will direct you to the Amazon reviews section.

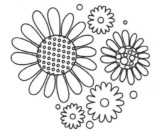

Thanks for adding a bit more color to the world!

Brissa Ocean

Made in United States
North Haven, CT
12 December 2024

62257116R00057